CONQUERING TEMPTATION

A value packed Journey to Overcoming Porn Addiction

Patrick Moore

Copyright@2023 Patrick Moore

This book is a work of nonfiction. Any resemblance to actual person, living or dead, or actual events is coincidental.

TABLE OF CONTENTS

INTRODUCTION

For many years, John struggled with porn addiction. Despite his best efforts to quit, he always found himself slipping back into old patterns. He felt ashamed, powerless, and hopeless. But one day, John made a decision that changed his life forever. He realized that in order to overcome his addiction, he needed to confront the root causes and make a concerted effort to change.

This is the story of John's journey to conquering temptation and reclaiming control over his life. Through his struggles and triumphs, John discovered powerful strategies for overcoming porn addiction and found the support and encouragement he needed to succeed. Whether you are just beginning your own journey, or have been struggling for years, "Conquering Temptation" will offer you the insights, tools, and hope you need to overcome your addiction and find a path towards lasting freedom.

CONQUERING TEMPTATION

CHAPTER 1

Understanding Porn Addiction

Definition and Symptoms

Porn addiction: What it is and how to recognize it

Porn addiction is characterized as a compulsive urge to view pornographic media despite its drawbacks. Porn addicts frequently spend a lot of time thinking about, viewing, and doing porn-related activities, which negatively impacts their relationships, careers, and social lives. Porn addiction symptoms can include excessive pornography viewing, spending a lot of time and money on porn, putting off chores to partake in pornographic activities, and feeling bad or humiliated after seeing porn. Other signs may include frequent masturbation, trouble building or sustaining close relationships, trouble resisting desires or cravings to watch porn, and feeling upset when unable to access porn.

Not everyone who watches porn is necessarily struggling with an addiction, it is vital to remember this. However, professional assistance can be required if a person's use of pornography is out of control and negatively affecting their lives.

Cognitive-behavioral therapy is frequently used to treat porn addiction since it focuses on assisting the patient in recognizing and altering problematic habits and thought patterns. Group therapy, medication, and lifestyle changes are among more therapeutic options.

It is crucial to seek assistance from a licensed mental health professional if you or someone you know is suffering from a porn addiction.

The Impact on Mental and Physical Health

Mental and physical health can both be impacted by stress. Mental health can be affected by stress in numerous ways, including increased anxiety, depression, and difficulty concentrating. Physical health can also be affected by stress, with symptoms such as headaches, muscle tension, and an increased risk of developing chronic illnesses. Stress can also lead to unhealthy coping behaviors, such as overeating or substance abuse. It is important to manage stress levels in order to maintain both physical and mental wellbeing.

There are a variety of techniques that can be used to reduce stress, including relaxation techniques such as meditation, exercise, and deep breathing. Taking time for yourself to do activities that you enjoy can also help reduce stress. Additionally, talking to a mental health professional can help to identify and address any underlying issues that may be contributing to stress.

Overall, it is important to be mindful of the impact that stress can have on mental and physical health, and to take steps to reduce stress in order to maintain overall wellbeing.

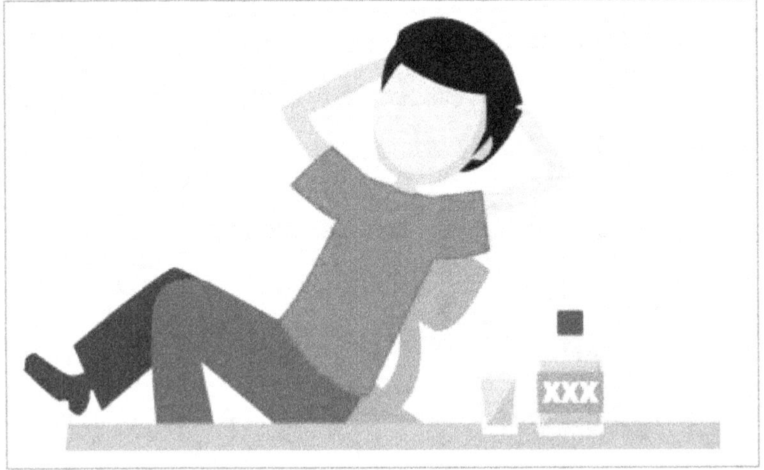

Common Misconceptions

1. **Porn addiction is a new phenomenon** – This is not true. Pornography has been around for centuries, and it is likely that people have become addicted to it for just as long.

2. **Porn addiction isn't a real addiction** – Porn addiction is a real psychological condition that can have serious consequences for those suffering from it.

3. **Porn addiction only affects men** – While it is true that the majority of people who struggle with pornography addiction are male, a growing number of women are also being affected by it.

4. **People who watch porn don't have a problem** – Not necessarily. Some people may be able to watch pornography without developing an addiction, but for others it can be an issue that requires professional help.

5. **Porn addiction only affects married people** – This is not true. Porn addiction can affect anyone regardless of marital status.

6. **Porn addiction can be cured by abstaining from porn** – While abstaining from porn is an important part of the recovery process, it is not a cure-all. Professional help may be necessary to fully address the underlying issues that are contributing to the addiction.

7. **Porn addiction is a moral issue** – Porn addiction is a mental health issue, not a moral one. People who struggle with porn addiction need to be treated with compassion, not judgment.

8. **Porn addiction is a sign of weakness** – Like any addiction, porn addiction is a sign of underlying issues that need to be addressed. It is not a sign of weakness or moral failing.

9. **Watching porn is harmless** – While it is true that not all pornography is dangerous, some of it can be quite harmful to those who watch it. It is important to be aware of the potential risks of viewing certain types of pornography.

10. **People who watch porn are perverts** – This is a very unfair and inaccurate stereotype. People who watch porn can be of any gender, age, or background. They should not be judged or labeled based on their viewing habits.

CHAPTER 2

The Root Causes of Porn Addiction

Personal Trauma

Personal trauma can be a cause of porn addiction, though the exact mechanisms of how this happens are not entirely clear. It is possible that people who have experienced trauma, such as abuse, neglect, or other forms of psychological distress, may turn to porn in order to escape these painful memories or experiences. Pornography can provide a temporary escape from reality, allowing them to forget their trauma and create a fantasy world in which they can control the outcome. In addition, the anonymity of the internet may make it easier for a person to access and view pornographic material without fear of judgement or stigma. The act of watching porn can also be associated with a pleasurable, if temporary, release of stress hormones, which may explain why a person may become addicted to this behavior. Finally, the repetitive nature of porn may serve as a form of self-medication, providing a form of distraction from the pain of the trauma.

In any case, it is important to recognize that trauma can be a contributing factor in an individual's struggle with porn addiction, and that treatment should be tailored to address the underlying issues as well as the addiction itself. Professional help can provide support for those struggling with both trauma and addiction, and can help an individual create healthy coping strategies to manage both.

In addition to seeking help from a professional, individuals may benefit from engaging in activities that promote healing from trauma and also provide a sense of connection and safety. Examples of activities that may be beneficial in healing from trauma include yoga, meditation, journaling, spending time in nature, and other forms of self-care. Finally, it is important to remember that recovery is possible and that with the right tools and support, individuals can recover from trauma and porn addiction.

Unmet Emotional Needs

Unmet emotional needs are one of the primary causes of porn addiction. Pornography can provide an escape from reality, allowing people to fulfill their emotional needs and desires in a fantasy world. This can lead to an unhealthy reliance on pornography as a coping mechanism that can lead to an addiction. Unmet emotional needs can include loneliness, a lack of satisfaction in relationships, low self-esteem, and a lack of purpose or direction in life. When these needs are not met, people turn to pornography in an attempt to fill the void.

Additionally, unresolved trauma and other psychological conditions can increase the risk of developing a porn addiction. People who have experienced trauma may use pornography as a way to cope with the pain and discomfort associated with the event. Additionally, people with mental health conditions, such as anxiety and depression, may use pornography as a distraction from their symptoms. This can lead to an unhealthy dependence on pornography as a way to manage emotions and feelings.

Finally, cultural influences can play a role in the development of porn addiction. Pornography is widely available and accepted as a form of entertainment, and it is often portrayed as a harmless activity. This can lead to a false sense of security and acceptance when viewing porn, which can lead to an addiction.

Chemical Imbalances

The cause of porn addiction is not definitively known but is thought to be related to various factors, including psychological, biological, and social. In particular, there is some evidence that suggests that chemical imbalances in the brain may contribute to porn addiction.

Neurochemical imbalances can cause someone to feel pleasure differently, which could make them more likely to engage in activities that provide a pleasurable effect. For instance, a person with an imbalance in dopamine, the neurotransmitter responsible for pleasure and reward, may be more prone to seeking out activities such as watching porn that produce a pleasurable effect. In addition, increased levels of the hormone cortisol, which is associated with stress and anxiety, may lead someone to turn to porn as a way of self-soothing or avoiding unpleasant emotions.

As with any addiction, it is important to seek professional help if you or someone you know is dealing with a porn addiction. A qualified mental health professional can help to identify the root causes of the addiction and develop an effective treatment plan.

Additionally, there are also a variety of self-help resources available, such as self-help books or online support groups, that can help someone struggling with porn addiction. If you or someone you know is struggling with porn addiction, it is important to take the necessary steps to get help and support.

In conclusion, while chemical imbalances may play a role in porn addiction, other factors such as psychological, biological, and social influences may also be involved. It is important to seek professional help to properly diagnose and treat porn addiction.

CHAPTER 3

Strategies for Overcoming Addiction

Mindfulness and Self-Awareness

Mindfulness and self-awareness are powerful tools to help you overcome porn addiction. Mindfulness helps you become aware of your thoughts and feelings, allowing you to take steps to change the behaviors that are causing the addiction. Self-awareness allows you to recognize your triggers and understand the underlying issues that are fueling the addiction.

When dealing with porn addiction, mindfulness can help you recognize when you're feeling the urge to watch porn. By becoming aware of your thoughts, you can pause and reflect on why you're feeling the urge. This can help you identify potential triggers and address the underlying issues behind the addiction.

Self-awareness is also key to overcoming porn addiction. This involves recognizing the patterns and behaviors that are contributing to your addiction. It also involves being honest with yourself about the way you're feeling and why you're struggling. This can help you identify the underlying triggers that are causing the addiction and take steps to address them.

In addition to these two practices, it can also be helpful to practice self-care and engage in activities that bring you joy and satisfaction. This can help to replace the negative behaviors of porn addiction with positive ones, allowing you to move away from the addiction in a healthier way.

Finally, it's important to reach out for help if you're struggling with porn addiction. Talking to a therapist or support group can help you process your emotions and find healthier ways of dealing with them. This can be an important step in overcoming the addiction and finding a healthier way of living.

By practicing mindfulness and self-awareness, you can take important steps toward overcoming your porn addiction. With the right tools and support, you can find freedom from addiction and lead a healthier life.

Identifying Triggers

Triggers for porn addiction can vary from person to person. Some common triggers may include negative emotions (such as loneliness, depression, or stress), boredom, feeling inadequate, relationship issues, feeling disconnected, or even positive emotions (such as excitement or anticipation). Other potential triggers can include environmental factors, such as seeing an attractive person or having access to pornography online. It can also be triggered by thoughts of past experiences with porn or even a desire to escape from reality.

The key to managing porn addiction is to identify and address the underlying triggers that contribute to the addiction. This can involve therapy, support groups, and lifestyle changes. It is also important to have a plan for when faced with a trigger, such as identifying a distraction or reaching out for help.

The best way to address porn addiction is to develop healthy coping strategies that can help to manage and reduce the urge to view porn. This can include developing healthier outlets for stress and negative emotions, such as exercise, creative outlets, or talking to a friend or therapist. Additionally, setting boundaries and avoiding high-risk situations can help to reduce the risk of relapse.

Finally, it is important to remember that recovery is possible and that it takes time and effort. Seeking professional help and support can be a great way to get started on the path to recovery.

Building Healthy Coping

1. **Practice mindfulness and self-awareness**: Mindfulness can be a powerful tool for managing porn addiction. Take time to practice mindfulness and observe your thoughts and feelings without judgment. This can help you identify triggers and gain clarity on the underlying causes of your addiction.

2. **Take breaks from technology**: Set limits on how often you allow yourself to access technology, such as smartphones and computers. This helps to reduce the temptation to access porn and other triggers.

3. **Exercise**: Exercise is a great way to release endorphins and reduce stress. Regular exercise can also help you manage feelings of anxiety, depression and low self-esteem that may be contributing to your porn addiction.

4. **Connect with supportive people**: Surround yourself with people who will support and encourage your recovery efforts. Having conversations about your struggles with trusted friends and family can help you gain perspective and build healthy coping skills.

5. **Seek professional help**: If your attempts to manage your porn addiction haven't been successful, it's important to seek professional help. A trained therapist can help you identify and address the underlying issues that contribute to your porn addiction and provide guidance on how to develop healthy coping mechanisms.

6. **Find healthy outlets**: Find healthy outlets to replace the need to view porn. Participate in activities that provide a sense of accomplishment and fulfillment, such as hobbies, volunteer work and sports.

7. **Practice self-care**: Take time to practice self-care and nourish your mind, body and soul. This might include getting enough sleep, eating nutritious meals, meditating and engaging in activities that bring you joy.

8. **Develop a support system**: Develop a support system of people to turn to when you feel the urge to watch porn. Talking to someone can help to distract you and provide motivation to stay on track.

9. **Use distraction techniques**: When you're feeling the urge to watch porn, distract yourself by doing something

else. This might include going for a walk, reading a book, or listening to music.

10. **Avoid triggers**: Avoid situations or activities that trigger the urge to watch porn. This might include spending time on social media, surfing the web, or watching movies.

11. **Develop positive affirmations**: Create positive affirmations and repeat them to yourself when you're feeling the urge to watch porn. This can help to reframe your thoughts and give you the motivation to stay on track.

12. **Reward yourself**: Celebrate small successes and reward yourself when you've made progress in managing your porn addiction. This will help to reinforce healthy behaviors and motivate you to continue with your recovery efforts.

13. **Practice gratitude**: Make time each day to be thankful for the things you have in your life. Practicing gratitude can help to reduce negative thoughts and keep you focused on the positive.

14. **Seek out meaningful relationships**: Work on building meaningful relationships with people who are supportive and understanding. This can help to reduce feelings of

isolation and loneliness that may be contributing to your porn addiction.

15. **Set goals**: Set realistic goals for yourself and work on achieving them. Having a sense of purpose can help to motivate you and provide a sense of accomplishment.

16. **Take time to reflect**: Reflection can be a powerful tool for managing porn addiction. Take time to reflect on your thoughts and feelings and identify any triggers or underlying issues that need to be addressed.

17. **Practice self-acceptance**: Work on accepting yourself and loving yourself unconditionally. Self-acceptance can help to reduce feelings of shame or guilt that may be contributing to your porn addiction

18. **Find ways to express yourself**: Find creative outlets to express yourself, such as music, writing, art, or dance. This can help to reduce feelings of stress and provide an emotional release.

19. **Take care of your physical health**: Make sure to get enough sleep, eat nutritious meals, and drink plenty of water. Taking care of your physical health can help to

reduce feelings of stress and anxiety that may be contributing to your porn addiction.

20. **Track your progress**: Track your progress and celebrate your successes. This can help to motivate you to stay on track and continue working on managing your porn addiction.

By implementing these healthy coping mechanisms, you can gain the strength and clarity you need to manage your porn addiction. With time and dedication, you can begin to develop healthier habits and live an addiction-free life.

Connecting with Support

If you or a loved one are struggling with porn addiction, there are a variety of resources available to help you. Seeking support from a qualified therapist or counselor is one of the most effective ways to address porn addiction. Professional help can provide an understanding, non-judgmental environment where you can discuss the underlying issues contributing to the addiction. Other resources include support groups such as Sex Addicts Anonymous and Sex and Love Addicts Anonymous, which offer peer-led support to those struggling with porn addiction. Additionally, online forums, such as NoFap, provide a safe space to discuss your journey and connect with individuals who are also trying to overcome porn addiction. Lastly, don't forget to reach out to your family and friends for social support.

No matter what resources you choose to use, know that you are not alone and recovery is possible.

CHAPTER 4

The Journey to Recovery

The Importance of Self-Care

Self-care is an essential component of recovery from porn addiction. Self-care helps to reduce stress and improve overall mental, physical, and emotional health. It also helps to provide a sense of control and positive coping skills, which can be extremely important in navigating the challenges that come with recovery from a porn addiction. Self-care can help to reduce feelings of shame and guilt, improve self-esteem, provide a sense of hope, and serve as an important tool for relapse prevention. Self-care activities can also help to rebuild healthy relationships and provide a sense of purpose and connection. Finally, self-care can help to create a pathway towards lasting recovery and build a foundation for a healthy and fulfilling life.

Whether it's through exercise, mindfulness, creative outlets, or spending time with friends, self-care should be a priority in any recovery plan. It can be easy to forget, but self-care is an important part of the recovery journey and can be a powerful tool in working towards a healthier and more fulfilling life.

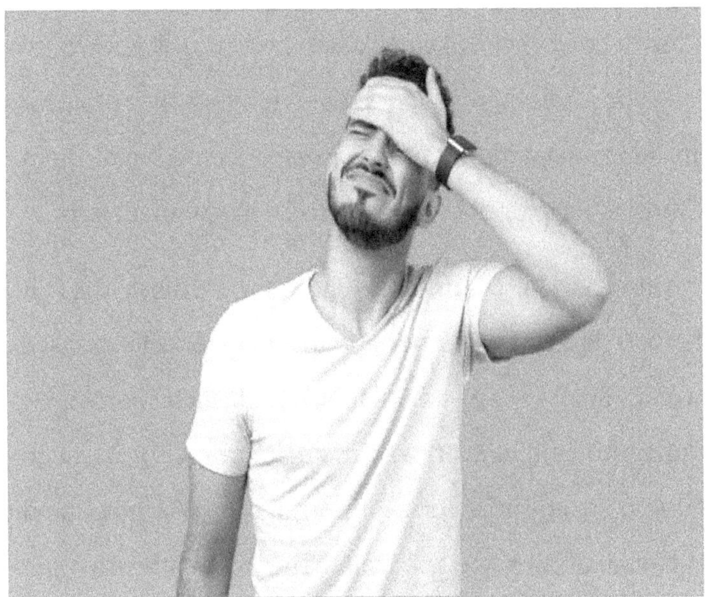

Dealing with Setbacks

1. **Acknowledge the Setback**: It's important to acknowledge when a setback has occurred, whether it is a relapse or a minor slip-up. Acknowledging the setback will help in understanding what caused it and can help in creating a plan for preventing it from happening again.

2. **Analyze the Setback**: Once the setback has been acknowledged, it is important to analyze what caused it. Was it due to an external trigger such as seeing a pornographic image or was it an internal trigger such as feeling a strong urge to view pornography? Understanding the cause of the setback can help in creating a plan to prevent it from happening again.

3. **Talk to Someone**: It is important to talk to someone about the setback. Talking to a trusted friend, family member, or therapist can be helpful in understanding the setback and can provide support in dealing with it.

4. **Develop a Plan**: Developing a plan to prevent similar setbacks from occurring in the future is important. This plan should include strategies to manage triggers, such as avoiding certain websites or situations, and should include

healthy coping strategies such as exercising or engaging in an activity that distracts from the urge to view pornography.

5. **Seek Professional Help**: If the setback is severe or if it occurs repeatedly, it may be beneficial to seek professional help. A therapist can provide additional support and guidance in dealing with the setback and can help develop a plan to prevent it from happening again.

6. **Stay Positive**: It is important to remember that setbacks are a normal part of recovery and that they don't mean that recovery is not possible. Staying positive and focusing on the progress that has been made can be helpful in dealing with setbacks.

7. **Move Forward**: Once the setback has been acknowledged and addressed, it is important to move forward and focus on the progress that has been made. It is important to forgive oneself and to start the recovery process again.

Recovering from porn addiction is a difficult process and setbacks can occur. It is important to acknowledge the setback, analyze what caused it, and develop a plan to prevent it from happening again. Additionally, seeking professional help and staying positive can be beneficial in dealing with the setback. Lastly, it is important to move forward and focus on the progress that has been made.

Recovering from porn addiction is possible, and it is important to remember that setbacks are a normal part of the process. With perseverance and dedication, it is possible to overcome porn addiction and to recover.

Staying Motivated

1. **Set realistic goals**. Setting unrealistic goals will make recovery seem impossible and can lead to feelings of discouragement and frustration. Aim to make small, achievable goals that will help you make progress in your recovery.

2. **Find a support system**. Find people who can understand and support you. Talking to other individuals who are going through the same thing can be incredibly motivating and beneficial.

3. **Take it one day at a time**. Don't focus too much on the long-term goal or the end result. Instead, focus on the present and take it one day at a time.

4. **Celebrate your successes**. Celebrating your successes, no matter how small they are, is a great start to stay motivated. Recognize when you make progress and reward yourself for it!

5. **Stay positive**. It can be hard to stay positive when you're struggling with addiction, but it's important to maintain a

positive attitude. Remind yourself that you can do this and that you are capable of making progress in your recovery.

6. **Make a plan for when you're feeling down**. When you're feeling discouraged or overwhelmed, make a plan for how to deal with it. This could include talking to a friend, going for a walk, or engaging in a hobby. Having a plan in place for when you're feeling down can help you stay motivated.

7. **Take care of yourself**. Make sure you're taking care of your physical, emotional, and mental health. Taking care of yourself will help you stay motivated and make progress in your recovery.

8. **Seek help**. If you feel like you need extra support, don't be afraid to seek help from a professional. A therapist, counselor, or other mental health professional can provide you with the support and guidance you need to stay on track with your recovery.

9. **Find activities that you enjoy**. Finding activities that you enjoy can help you stay motivated and focused on your recovery. Try to find activities that can help you relax and

that you enjoy doing. This could be anything from taking a walk to reading a book.

10. **Avoid triggers**. This can be difficult, but it's important to avoid any situations or people that may trigger your addiction. Whenever possible, try to stay away from triggers in order to stay motivated and on track with your recovery.

Recovery from porn addiction can be difficult, but it is possible. By setting realistic goals, finding a support system, taking it one day at a time, and staying positive, you can stay motivated and make progress in your recovery.

Celebrating Progress

1. **Celebrate each day of sobriety**. Break the habit of viewing pornography by setting a goal of one week, one month, or longer of sobriety. Make sure you take the time to appreciate the progress you are making and the willpower you are demonstrating.

2. **Reward yourself for making progress**. Give yourself something to look forward to when you complete a certain goal. This could be an outing with friends, a massage, a new item of clothing, or anything else that you can afford and enjoy.

3. **Celebrate the small victories**. Each day of sobriety and each step towards recovery is an accomplishment. Take the time to reflect on how far you have come and how much closer you are to reaching your goals.

4. **Celebrate with friends and family**. Recovery from porn addiction is a journey that you do not have to face alone. Celebrate your progress with your loved ones and share the joy of overcoming such a challenge.

5. **Make a commitment to yourself**. Make a promise to yourself that you are going to stay the course and continue to make progress on your journey to recovery. This will help you in staying motivated and focused on your goals.

6. **Take time for self-care**. Make sure to set aside some time each day to practice self-care. This could include activities like yoga, meditation, journaling, or reading. Taking care of yourself is an important part of recovery and should be celebrated.

7. **Celebrate with a treat**. Go out for a special meal or treat yourself to an indulgence to celebrate the progress you have made in recovery. This will help you feel good and remind you of the progress you are making.

8. **Celebrate with a meaningful activity**. Spend time doing something that is important to you or that you enjoy. This could be something like going for a walk, playing an instrument, or painting. Doing something meaningful can be a great way to celebrate and can help keep you motivated on your path to recovery.

By celebrating the progress you are making in your recovery from porn addiction, you will be able to stay motivated and focused on your goals. With daily reflection, self-care, and rewards, you can celebrate each step on your journey.

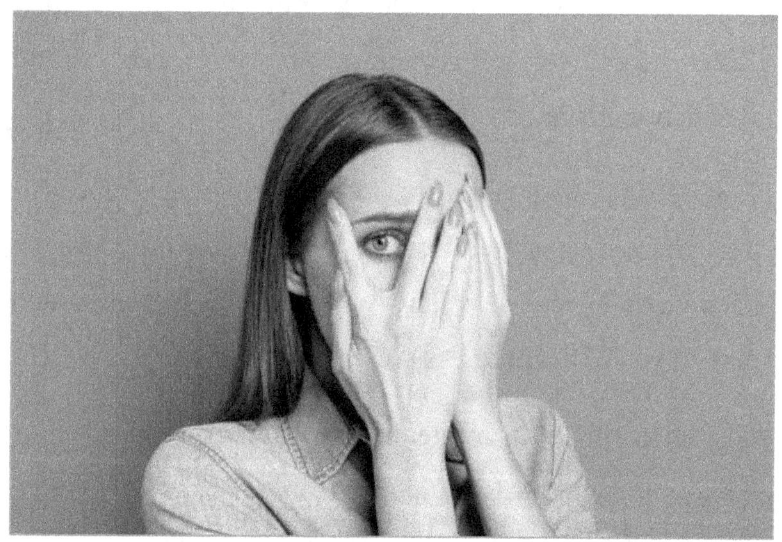

CHAPTER 5

Moving Forward: Life after Addiction

Maintaining Sobriety

It can be difficult to beat a porn addiction, but staying sober after recovery is just as crucial. Here are some pointers for staying sober:

Create a solid network of support: Surround yourself with understanding and eager to assist you in staying on track friends and family.

Recognize your pornographic urges' triggers, then devise a strategy to deal with or prevent them.

Find substitute activities: Take up new hobbies, interests, or volunteer work to occupy the time that was previously spent watching porn.

Seek therapy: To assist you in resolving underlying emotional difficulties and preserving your sobriety, think about visiting a therapist or joining a support group.

Keep yourself on track and accountable by checking in with a reliable friend or accountability partner on a regular basis.

It takes time and work to overcome a porn addiction, but with dedication and assistance, it is possible to stay sober and have a full life.

Building a Fulfilling Life

To build a fulfilling life after porn addiction, consider the following steps:

Seek professional help: A therapist or counselor can help you understand the root causes of your addiction and provide guidance for recovery.

Build a support network: Surround yourself with friends and family who will support you in your journey towards recovery.

Replace negative habits with positive ones: Focus on developing new interests and hobbies that bring joy and fulfillment to your life.

Practice self-care: Take care of your physical, emotional, and mental well-being by exercising, eating well, and getting enough sleep.

Stay accountable: Keep track of your progress and seek accountability from others to help stay on track.

Stay away from triggers: Avoid people, places, and activities that trigger your addiction.

Cultivate healthy relationships: Focus on building meaningful relationships with others and avoid toxic ones.

Remember, recovery is a journey and it takes time and effort. Be patient with yourself and stay focused on your goals.

Overcoming Relapse

To overcome relapse when recovering from porn addiction, consider the following steps:

Identify triggers: Recognize the events, emotions, and situations that trigger your urge to watch porn.

Have a plan in place: Develop a plan for how you will deal with triggers when they arise. This might include calling a friend, engaging in physical activity, or seeking support from a support group.

Build resilience: Develop healthy coping mechanisms and resilience to stress, so you are better equipped to deal with difficult emotions and situations.

Surround yourself with support: Seek support from friends, family, or a therapist who can provide you with encouragement and accountability.

Seek professional help: If necessary, consider seeking professional help from a therapist or counselor who specializes in treating porn addiction.

Stay accountable: Regularly check in with someone you trust to help keep you accountable and to discuss any challenges you may be facing.

Practice self-reflection: Regularly reflect on your thoughts and feelings, and identify any patterns that may contribute to your urge to watch porn.

Remember, overcoming relapse takes time and effort. Stay committed to your recovery and don't be afraid to seek help when you need it.

CONCLUSION

Encouragement to Continue the Journey

Overcoming addiction is a challenging journey, but it's important to remember that you are not alone and that it's possible to break free from the cycle of addiction. Here are some tips to help you stay motivated:

Set clear goals: Define what you want to achieve and make a plan to reach those goals. This will give you a sense of direction and purpose also.

Find support: Talk to friends and family, seek support from a therapist, or join a support group for those struggling with addiction. Having a supportive network also helps.

Educate yourself: Learn as much as you can about addiction and the strategies that have worked for others in overcoming it. This will give you a better understanding of what you're facing and equip you with tools to help you succeed.

Practice self-care: Taking care of yourself physically, emotionally, and mentally is crucial in overcoming addiction. Exercise, eat well, get enough sleep, and engage in activities that bring you joy and peace.

Recognize and challenge negative thoughts: Addiction can be accompanied by negative thoughts and self-doubt. Challenge these thoughts and focus on your goals, strengths, and progress.

Remember that overcoming addiction takes time and effort, but with persistence and dedication, you can succeed. Stay positive and keep pushing forward.

A Final Note of Hope

It's important to remember that overcoming porn addiction is a journey and not a destination. There will be setbacks and challenges, but it's important to stay motivated and keep pushing forward. Keep in mind that it's normal to stumble, but it's not okay to give up. With every small victory, you are one step closer to breaking free from addiction.

Remember that you are not defined by your addiction, and that it's never too late to change. With hard work, dedication, and the right support, you can overcome porn addiction and reclaim control over your life. So stay strong, stay focused, and never give up hope. You are capable of achieving greatness and living a life free from addiction.